Start Here

a guide for parents of autistic kids

The Autistic Press
WASHINGTON, DC

Brought to you by:
Autistic Self Advocacy Network
Autistic Women & Nonbinary Network
Little Lobbyists
Thinking Person's Guide to Autism

Contents

Forward

Two months before our younger child's fourth birthday, my husband and I learned that she is autistic. Her hours-long evaluation at one of the best research centers in the world was not her first assessment for autism, just the first that resulted in a diagnosis. In one sense, after a year and a half of wondering, it came as a relief to know for certain; to be given a definitive answer, instead of the well-intentioned reassurances of our family doctor—who didn't believe our daughter was autistic—or the "on the fence" musings of the last developmental specialist we'd seen.

But we were also hoping for practical guidance, information about how to best help and support our child. The doctor spoke to us for about ten minutes after delivering the news, printed out some website content we could have easily found on our own, recommended speech therapy (which our child was already receiving), and sent us on our way. There was nothing in the way of advice or encouragement; no one acknowledged our child's strengths, or suggested how we might help her build on them. I'll never forget how lost and anxious I felt as we drove home with our daughter snoozing in her carseat—not because of the diagnosis, which we'd already suspected, but because we were still effectively clueless and empty-handed.

This booklet is the resource I wish we'd been given then.

I've been where you are as the parent of a newly diagnosed autistic child, or one wondering if your child might be autistic. I know the most important thing to you, as a parent, is determining how to best help and support your child. The single most valuable piece of advice I can offer to any parent of an autistic child is to listen to autistic adults. Autistic people are the experts on autism. As a parent in a neuroatypical family, I am so grateful for ASAN's work, their resources, and their advocacy. Like all of their materials, this parent booklet is clear, factual, well-researched, and accessible. And it is the work of an autistic community my child and yours will one day have access to.

It's been years since my child's diagnosis, yet the things I most want for her have not changed: the education and support she is entitled to, the opportunities she wants, the acceptance she deserves. I want her to be seen and respected and valued for who she is. I want her to feel and be empowered. The work of ASAN is one thing that makes me hope and believe all these things are possible.

Your child is autistic. So is mine. They have been all along; remember that this diagnosis changes nothing about who they are. Your kid is the same kid you have always known and loved. And they are exactly who they are meant to be.

— *Nicole Chung, author and parent*

ONE

To Start

If you're reading this, your child probably just received an autism diagnosis. For some parents, you might not have expected this news. For other parents, you may have wondered if your child is autistic. Either way, you probably noticed ways that your child seems different from other kids. Autism is a way to explain what those differences are and why they happen.

Your kid is still the same kid as they were before they got their autism diagnosis. All the things you love about them haven't changed. Your kid loves you, and they know you love them. Now that you know that they are autistic, you are going to be able to understand them better.

Being autistic is a part of what makes your child who they are. Autism doesn't mean that your child will have a worse life than other children. Their life may be different than what you had expected. But your child can still have a great life. Part of building that great life for your child is learning how to support them as an autistic person. We hope this booklet can help you learn how to do that.

When you hear the word "autism", it usually isn't talked about in a good way. The way that doctors and the media talk about autism can be scary. A lot of what people say they know about autism is wrong. So you might be scared or confused about your child and their future. That's okay. We'll tell you the facts about autism in this booklet. Autism is nothing to be afraid of.

But right now, know that you have already done great work to support your child. Now that you know they are autistic, you can use that information to help your child. You can help them learn and grow.

You can also learn and grow with them! You can learn more about the autistic community. Autistic adults are here to teach you more about autism. Many of us are also parents of autistic children. We will let you know how you can connect to autistic people in your community.

This booklet was written by autistic adults, along with parents of autistic children. Autistic adults used to be autistic kids ourselves. That means we can offer important information about autism that doctors or others might miss. Because autistic people are the main authors, when we talk about autistic people in this booklet, we will use first-person pronouns (we, us, ours). We believe that autistic people are experts when it comes to autism. If you want to learn more about autism, you should always start by listening to autistic people.

We're excited to share what we know about autism with you. We know that this can be a lot of information to take in. It's okay if you aren't ready to read the rest of this booklet right now. It's okay if you need to take a break. You can also read this booklet one section at a time, or talk through what you read with a loved one. We will be here when you are ready.

What is autism?

It's important to know that your child didn't "become" autistic. Research shows that children are born autistic. They will always be autistic. It may have been harder to notice they were autistic when they were a baby. Most babies look and act the same way. That's why most autistic kids get diagnosed when they are a toddler or older.

Your child probably got diagnosed as autistic by a doctor. Someone can be autistic even if they don't get a diagnosis from a doctor. Because of myths about autism, it can be harder for some kinds of autistic people to get diagnoses. These groups are autistic adults, autistic girls, and autistic people of color. But anyone can be autistic, no matter what race, gender, or age.

Every autistic person experiences autism differently, but there are things that we all have in common. It's okay if your child doesn't experience everything on this list. There are lots of different ways to be autistic. That is okay!

1. **Autistic people think differently.** We may have very strong interests in very specific things. Your child might be able to talk for hours about dinosaurs, or spend a lot of time learning to draw maps. They might love to stare at the washing machine, or line things up. We might be great problem-solvers, or pay close attention to detail.

   It might take us longer to think about things. For example, it may take your child a longer time to answer a question. We might have trouble organizing our thoughts. That can make it harder to figure out how to start and finish a task, or make decisions.

   Routines are important for many autistic people. It can be hard for us to deal with surprises or unexpected changes.

Sticking to a schedule can be helpful. Your child might want to eat the same food every day, or always watch tv at the same time.

When we get overwhelmed, we might not be able to process our thoughts, feelings, and surroundings. That can cause us to have meltdowns, which can make us lose control of our body. For your child, this might look like a tantrum, but they are not the same thing, and should not be treated the same way. We will talk about that more later.

2. **We process our senses differently.** Your child might be extra sensitive to things like bright lights or loud sounds. We might have trouble understanding what we hear or what our senses tell us. We might not notice if we are in pain or hungry.

   Because our senses are so sensitive, the world can be overwhelming to autistic people. To help process sensory information, we might do the same movement over and over again. This is called "stimming". For example, your child might rock back and forth, flap their hands, or hum. This can help us feel calm, help us pay attention, or just feel good. Stimming is an important part of being autistic. You should make sure your child is allowed to stim.

3. **We move differently.** A lot of autistic people feel like our bodies don't always listen to our brains. Your child might have trouble with fine motor skills or coordination. They might walk in a way that looks a little bit different from other people. They might seem "clumsy", or have bad handwriting. It can also be hard for us to start or stop moving. For example, your child might have trouble

getting up to come for dinner. It might take them longer to stand up, even if they want to.

Because autism affects movement, it can affect speech. When we speak, we move our lips, tongue, throat, and lots of other things at the same time. So, autistic people might not be able to control how loud our voices are. We might speak in a monotone, or in a sing-song voice. Or, we might not be able to speak at all. It's important to know that even if an autistic person can't speak, we can usually understand what other people say.

4. **We communicate differently.** We process language differently. We might take a while to understand and respond to things people say to us. We might also understand things differently. For example, your child might not know if someone is joking, even if your child knows how to tell jokes. Or, they might take things literally.

   We also use words differently. We might have a different sense of humor. We might talk using echolalia (repeating things we have heard before). If you notice your child repeating a line they heard on TV, that is echolalia. It is a way we try to communicate, even if other people might not understand what we mean. Over time, you can learn what your child means when they use echolalia.

   Autistic kids often start talking later than other kids. We might also learn to talk more slowly. If your autistic child is not speaking yet, they might just be getting ready. In the meantime, there are ways to communicate without speaking. Your child is already trying to communicate with you, whether or not they can speak.

Some autistic people use Augmentative and Alternative Communication (AAC) to communicate. For example, we may communicate by typing on a computer, or pointing to pictures on an iPad. Some people may also communicate with behavior or the way we act. For example, your child might run away if you try and take them somewhere they don't want to go. Not every autistic person can talk, but we all have important things to say.

If your child doesn't talk, they can use AAC. We will talk more later about using AAC to communicate.

5. **We socialize differently.** Some of us might not understand or follow social rules that non-autistic people made up. We might be more blunt or to-the-point than other people. Your child might be very honest. But other people might think they are being rude, even if they don't mean to be.

Eye contact might make us uncomfortable. Your child might not look at you when you talk to them. But that doesn't mean they aren't listening. We also might have a hard time controlling our body language or facial expressions. That can confuse non-autistic people and make it harder to socialize.

Some of us might not be able to guess how people feel. Your child might not be able to tell if you're feeling happy or sad. Your child still cares how you feel! But they may not be able to tell from your face or your voice. They may need you to tell them how you are feeling instead.

Autistic people might have a hard time making friends. But that doesn't mean we don't want friends. Autistic kids may need help communicating with their peers. And their peers may need help communicating with them! The way autistic people socialize isn't bad. It's just different. We can have close friendships and be great friends, while still being ourselves.

There is no one way to be autistic. Some autistic people can speak, and some autistic people need to communicate in other ways. Some autistic people need a lot of help in our day-to-day lives, and some autistic people only need a little help. All of us are autistic, because there is no right or wrong way to be autistic. Every autistic person experiences autism differently. But we are all an important part of the world, and should be understood and accepted.

Autism and other disabilities

A lot of times, autistic kids aren't just autistic. Some disabilities happen more in autistic people, and autistic people usually have more than one disability. We might have other disabilities, like:

- Intellectual disabilities

- Mental health disabilities

- Learning disabilities

- ADHD

- Epilepsy

You might have found out when your child got their autism diagnosis that they also have other disabilities. Or, as your kid grows up, you might find out that they have other disabilities. There is lots of information out there about how to support autistic people with other disabilities. We will put some resources about that at the end of this booklet.

Sometimes, people say that because autistic people usually have other disabilities, that means autism is a bad thing. But that doesn't make sense. Think of it like this:

People with red hair sunburn more easily. Sunburns hurt and can cause skin cancer, but we don't say that red hair is bad. We don't try to cure red hair, or tell people with red hair to dye their hair. That wouldn't help with their sunburns. Instead, we make sure people wear sunblock.

It's the same with autism. Autistic people should get support for all of our needs. That includes supports for other disabilities, if we have any. We'll talk more about that later.

Sometimes, autistic people don't get an autism diagnosis. We might get diagnosed with the wrong disability instead. This might have happened to your child before.

Girls and people of color get the wrong diagnosis the most. When doctors first studied autism, they only looked at autistic white boys. Even today, doctors are less likely to think girls and people of color are autistic. They might get diagnosed with other disabilities instead, like intellectual disabilities or mental health disabilities.

What causes autism?

We don't know exactly what causes autism, but we know that it is genetic. You might not have another family member with an autism diagnosis from a doctor. But your child probably is not the only autistic person in your family. Many autistic people have lots of autistic family members. Even if you don't have any other autistic relatives, genes can change or be passed down in different ways. Genetics are complicated!

There is no cure for autism. Autism is not a disease. Autism is how our brains work. Autism doesn't make you sick, and you can't die from autism. Doctors can't stop us from being autistic. We don't "get better." We are okay being autistic. We are autistic our whole lives, and that is just how we are!

People usually want a cure for diseases. But most autistic people don't want a cure for autism. The goal of a cure is to 'fix' something, and autistic people don't need to be fixed.

Vaccines do not cause autism. In 1997, a man named Andrew Wakefield lied and said that vaccines caused autism. Lots of scientists proved him wrong. Vaccines do not cause autism. It is important to vaccinate your children so they don't get or spread dangerous diseases.

There is no autism "epidemic". People say that there are more autistic people now than there used to be. This is not true! In the year 2000, doctors said that about 1 in 150 people were autistic. Right now, they think 1 in 54 people are autistic. This isn't because more autistic people are being born. It's because doctors are getting better at diagnosing autistic people. Autistic people have always existed, but we get diagnosed more now than ever before. This is a good thing!

You did not cause your child's autism. Your child was born autistic. Nothing you did as a parent "made" your child autistic. If someone tells you that you made your child autistic, they are confused about how autism works. Or, they're just being a jerk!

What does an autism diagnosis mean for my kid?

You now know about an important part of what makes your child who they are. This is a great first step to making sure your child has the best life possible!

Your child may grow up to be different from what you expected. Their path through life may be different than other children's. Your child might need more support from family, friends, and their community. They might need help to learn how to live their life in the way that works best for them. That's okay! Your child can have a full and happy life. There is no limit on how good your child's life can be.

Some doctors might try and tell you what your child's future will look like. They might say your child will never talk, or live on their own. But there's no way of knowing what the future holds for your child. Lots of autistic people learn new skills later in life. They may be able to do things that others thought were impossible. Even if your child always needs a lot of help, they can still be in charge of their life. They will still be loved. They can still learn, work, and have fun. They still have a bright future ahead of them.

There may be certain things your child will never be able to do, and that's okay. But if a doctor tries to tell you what those things are now, they are lying. Over time, you'll learn more about your child. You'll figure out together what your child can do and wants to do. You can help them be the best they can be.

Some doctors might tell you that your child is "high-functioning" or "low-functioning". Try not to use these labels. When autistic people are called "low-functioning," people don't expect us to do well. When we are called "high-functioning," people think we don't need help to do well. Either way, we might not get the help we need. Functioning labels like these limit autistic people. You don't want to limit your child.

We like to use the words "support needs" instead. Support needs are just things autistic people need help with. Different autistic people need help with different things. Instead of using labels that don't help, just explain what your child can do. Explain what they need help with.

There is a lot to look forward to in your child's future. Just by learning that your child is autistic, you are already on the right track. As you learn more about autism, you will start to see more and more possibilities.

Should I treat my kid differently now?

Yes and no. Your child is still the same child as before they got an autism diagnosis. They still have the same personality, likes and dislikes. You should still treat your child with the same love and respect as you did before.

At the same time, now that you know your child is autistic, there are lots of things you can do to support them. Your support can help your child have an easier time in the world. Here are some things you can do to help support your child:

- Give them the tools to help manage their senses. This can be things as simple as giving them earplugs or headphones to deal with loud noises, or sunglasses to deal with bright lights. Notice what sensory situations upset your child, and work to fix those situations. For example, if your child has a hard time when they are in the living room, it could be that the light there is too bright. You could try turning off the light or switching to a less bright lightbulb to see if that helps.

- Understand that a meltdown is not the same as a tantrum. Meltdowns happen when autistic people get overwhelmed by our senses. We may get overwhelmed by things that don't bother you, like the noise of an air conditioner. That can make us lose control of our body.

  We can't control if or when we have a meltdown. We don't have meltdowns to try and get attention or get our way. If your child has a meltdown, never treat it like a tantrum. Never try to punish them, or say they are in trouble. That will probably make the meltdown worse! Give your child space to work through their feelings. Help them figure out what is overwhelming them. Work together to figure out what they can do about it.

  Having a meltdown is a difficult experience for autistic people. Treating your child with respect and care when meltdowns happen can make them a little easier. Over time, with your support, your child will learn more coping skills.

- Help your child communicate. Speech can be difficult for autistic people. But we still want to show others what we want and need. Working with a speech therapist can help make speech easier for some autistic people.

  Some autistic people can't talk at all. We can use things like sign language or pictures to say what we think. This is called Augmentative and Alternative Communication (AAC). Lots of autistic people use programs on tablets as their AAC. There are programs that pair words and pictures together. When your child touches the picture, the tablet says the word out loud. Your child can use the program to combine words into sentences and tell you what they think.

Some autistic people can talk sometimes, but not all of the time. If your kid can only talk sometimes, AAC is an important tool to have. It makes sure your child always has a way to communicate that works for them. Some people say AAC can keep children from learning to talk. They say that kids won't try to talk if they always have AAC. This is not true! Studies show that AAC can actually help some kids learn to talk.

We will have more resources on AAC at the end of this booklet.

- Help other people understand your child when they communicate. For example, your child might repeat a line from a movie when they are hungry. But the line from the movie seems to have nothing to do with being hungry. You can let other people know that your child is hungry when they say the movie line.

  You spend the most time with your child. That means that, besides your child, you probably understand best what your child is trying to say. Help other people in your life understand how your child communicates and what they are saying.

- Stick to routines with your child. Having structure helps your child get by in a world that can feel chaotic and confusing. Try to keep daily activities, like eating, bedtime, homework time, and free time, at the same times each day. You can create a daily schedule with pictures for your child. That way, they know what each day has in store for them. They have time to think through any changes in their routine.

- Some autistic people have a lot of trouble understanding spoken words. It can help to use pictures as much as possible: at home, at school, and everywhere else. Using a daily schedule that has pictures is one way to do this. For example, when you tell your child it is time to brush their teeth, you can also show them a picture of a child (or of them!) brushing their teeth. If your child has a hard time telling you what they want to do, you could show them pictures of different things to do. You can let them choose one of the pictures to show what they want to do.

  Social stories can also be a good tool. This is when you use pictures and text to explain to your child something that will happen. These can be helpful when doing something your child hasn't done before. For example, if your child needs to go see a new doctor, you can make them a social story. You can have pictures of the doctor, the doctor's office, and what will happen at the doctor's.

- Give your child time to process. This can mean a lot of different things! When talking to your child, it may take them longer to figure out how to answer. It might take a lot of energy for them to think through what someone else is saying. It can be hard to come up with what to say. Don't rush your child or interrupt them.

  Giving your child time to process also means letting your child know information about their lives as soon as you can. That way, they have enough time to think it through. It may take extra time for your child to adjust to a new routine, or to get used to doing something they have never done before. We talked about using social stories as a tool to help with this. It is much better for your child to know a change will happen beforehand. Changing something on short notice could make your child overwhelmed, or cause a meltdown.

- Let your child know that it is okay to be autistic. It is difficult to be autistic in a world that was not made for us. Many people don't understand autism. They might treat autistic people badly because of who we are. Your child may already think autism is bad. They may have heard that in school, from your family, or from their peers. Being positive about autism lets your child know that they can be themselves. It shows your child they can be proud of who they are.

  This also means that you need to find chances for your child to safely be who they are. Many autistic people face violence because they are autistic. Autistic people of color also face extra violence because of racism. For example, autistic people of color who stim in public may get targeted by police.

  There may be times that your child has to hide parts of who they are. That is part of staying safe as an autistic person. That's why it is so important that you find places for your child to be openly autistic. Your home should always be one of these places. You should also look for other chances for your child to be accepted for who they are.

Knowing about your child's autism should change how you treat your child in many ways. But there are also a lot of things that should stay the same. Your child is still the same kid that they were before they got diagnosed with autism. That means you should still treat your child like any other child their age. Remember that your kid is still a kid. Autism doesn't make your child less of a person.

Presuming competence

You should also always presume competence for your child. Sometimes, autistic people don't show what we think or know in ways that other people understand. Presuming competence means knowing that your child has thoughts and feelings. It means knowing that your child can understand and learn new things. You might not always be able to tell. But you should still treat your child with respect.

Remember that your child might use their behavior to show you how they think and feel. If your child is having a hard time with something, try and figure out how you can support them. Maybe they are in pain. Maybe the labels on their clothes are itchy. Don't assume they are acting out for no reason.

For a lot of parents, it can be hard to tell whether or not their child is paying attention. Some people feel very sure that their child is never listening. They think their kid doesn't understand anything they say. This can be scary! Some people get into the habit of talking about their kid in front of them. They assume their kid does not understand them. So they say bad things about their kid while their kid is there.

But many autistic adults remember hearing our parents say bad things about us. Our parents thought we couldn't listen or understand what they said. This can be a very sad and scary experience for a kid to have. It can harm their self-esteem, and make it harder for them to trust or connect with people.

You might be wrong about what your child does and doesn't understand. You could hurt them when you say bad things about them or autism in front of them.

On the other hand, what if you assume your child does understand? What if you're careful about what you say in front of them? Your child will notice your respect and love when you say good things. And even if they can't understand what you said, they won't get hurt by it. That's why it's always better to assume that your child is paying attention to what is happening. If they are around, avoid saying things that you wouldn't want them to hear.

Presuming competence also means having high expectations for your child. Your child has the potential to live a happy and full life. That potential hasn't changed because of getting an autism diagnosis. If your child shows interest in doing something, you should help them explore that interest. You should help even if others say it would be too difficult for your child to participate. Work to make sure that your child gets the same opportunities as other kids their age.

Your child may not be able to do *everything* that a non-autistic child can do. But that doesn't mean that they can't do *anything* that other children do. There may be things that only your child can do! For example, your child might not be able to write a story. But she might be great at word searches, or he might be the best artist in his class.

Having high expectations for your child also means making sure your child is included in society. That means living alongside people without disabilities. Your child should be in the same schools and social groups as non-disabled kids. When they get older, they should be in the same jobs and housing as people without disabilities. Autism does not mean that your child needs to be kept separate from everyone else. Even though some doctors, teachers, and other people might say so, this isn't true! We know that autistic people learn more and live better lives when we get to live and learn with everyone else. Fight for your child's right to be included!

What should I do next?

First off, take a deep breath. We know this is a lot of new information about your child and their life. Remember that your kid is still the same kid they were before they got an autism diagnosis. Having a diagnosis doesn't change who your kid is. It just helps explain why they might act or feel in certain ways.

Learning more about autism

The next thing you should do is learn more about autism. You are already doing this! We have explained a little about autism in this booklet. But there are lots of other sources that can give you more details.

It's important to know what sources about autism are good and what ones are bad. The best sources about autism come from autistic people ourselves! We are the experts when it comes to being autistic. There are lots of books and websites about autism written by autistic people.

Autism organizations can also be a good place to learn about autism. Autism organizations might have resources online or groups near you where you can go to learn more. There are some things you should look out for when seeing if an autism organization is a good resource for you:

- Make sure the organization listens to the voices of autistic people. They should have autistic people taking the lead in the group or on projects.

- Make sure the organization doesn't want to find a "cure" for autism. Remember, autism is just the way your child's brain works. Groups that look for a "cure" often tell parents to try dangerous things that can hurt your child. Some places even say you can "cure" autism by drinking bleach. Don't listen to organizations like these.

- Make sure the organization doesn't make autism seem like a scary or bad thing. Autism organizations should support your child. They should fight for a world where autistic people are included and treated fairly.

For example:

One bad autism organization is Autism Speaks. Most of their money goes towards doing research about autism. But, this research focuses on trying to make autistic people be "less autistic". This hurts autistic people. They don't spend a lot of money to help autistic people and our families. They have very few autistic people on their staff or board. Autism Speaks is not a good source to learn about autism.

One good autism organization is the Autistic People of Color Fund. They give money to help autistic people of color. They help people of color meet their own goals. They are run by autistic people.

At the end of this booklet, there is a list of some sources to learn about autism. Those are a good starting point for you to learn more.

Getting to know autistic adults

Another great way to learn about autism is meeting autistic adults. You can connect with autistic adults online. You can find local autism groups to meet autistic adults in-person. For parents, getting to know autistic adults can help you learn more about autism. You can get suggestions about what your child may be experiencing or ways to help them, see what is possible for them as they grow up, and more!

It's great to try and learn more from autistic adults. But not every autistic adult will want to talk about their life in a lot of detail with a stranger. Sometimes we just want to live our lives. That's okay! You should respect their privacy. There will be other chances to learn more.

Meeting autistic adults is also important for your child. Having autistic mentors is a way to show your child that being autistic is okay, and that they don't have to worry about growing up autistic. Getting to know other autistic people can give your child the chance to be themselves. It can help them learn tools that work for other autistic people. It can help them imagine what their future might look like.

TWO

All About Services

There are lots of different kinds of services for autistic people. These services can teach your child skills like:

- different ways to communicate

- motor skills, like handwriting or tying shoes

- how to do some daily life activities, like cooking or getting dressed

When we talk about autism services, we do not mean therapies specifically *for* autism. There is no therapy that will change autism. Some therapies will say that they can make your child less autistic. Newer studies show this is not true.

Remember: it's okay for your kid to be autistic! Even if you teach your child to hide their autism, they will still be autistic. But teaching us to hide our autism hurts us. It tells us that who we are isn't okay. It doesn't let us process our thoughts and feelings in ways that work for us. It makes our lives harder.

Services should help your autistic child live their best life as an autistic person. They should not try and make them non-autistic. You want your kid to be happy and have a good life. You want them to be able to be themselves, be in charge of their lives, and be included. They can be all of those things and still be autistic.

Good services help with specific needs your child has because they are autistic. They can help your child learn, grow, and communicate more easily. These services usually focus on specific skills, like communication, motor skills, or daily living. Good services should look at your child, their strengths, and what they need help with. They will work with you and your child to set goals that make sense for your child.

What services are out there?

- Services to help your child communicate. Some autistic people can speak, but have trouble being understood. They may speak very quickly or slowly, or pronounce words differently. Speech therapy can help with this. It can teach your child new words, and how to speak more clearly. It can help your child learn different ways to communicate.

  There are also services to help your child communicate even if they can't speak. Augmentative and Alternative Communication (AAC) are tools that your child can use to communicate without talking. These can be using picture cards, typing on a device like an iPad, using sign language, and more! All of these kinds of communication could work for your child. Service providers can help you try each of these to see what works best for your child. The service provider can help your child learn to use AAC, and how to make sentences. They can help your child learn to say all the different things they want to say.

- Services that help your child have more control over their body. Autistic people can struggle with gross motor skills (like walking and coordination). Physical therapy can help us learn these skills. Having your child do a physical activity, like swimming, martial arts, or dancing, can also help improve motor skills and be fun! It can also help your child feel calm in their body.

- Occupational therapy. This is a kind of service that can do many different things. It can help your child with fine motor skills (like writing or tying shoes). It can give your child tools to deal with their senses, so they are less overwhelmed. And, it can help your child learn independent living skills. They can learn how to take care of their daily hygiene, how to cook, and more!

- Services that help us learn to process our thoughts and feelings. A lot of autistic people have anxiety, because the world can be so overwhelming. We might also have trouble figuring out how we feel. A therapist can give your child strategies that can help.

  Many therapists focus on skills to make people seem less autistic. Make sure to avoid these therapists. Be sure to do extra research before choosing a therapist.

- Respite care services. Everyone needs a break sometimes. Respite is not just a break for your or your family - it is also a break for your child! It gives each of you some time to socialize separately. It lets you both recharge before getting back to your everyday life.

- Services that teach your child how to support themselves, or how you can support them. A service provider can help to make things more accessible for your child. For example, some autistic people have a hard time remembering what to do every day. The service provider can help your child use reminders on their phone. There are lots of strategies to make things easier for your child!

Once you figure out strategies for your child, you can tell others about them. You can work with other people that support your child, like teachers. You can get supports put into place wherever your child goes.

How do I know if services are good or bad?

There are a lot of different kinds of services out there. Some autism services are better than others. There are some kinds of services that can hurt autistic people. Every service and every service provider is different. So it is hard to say if any one type of service is "good" or "bad". You will need to look carefully at everyone who works with your child. Here are some things you should think about when looking at services:

- Does the service try to make your child seem less autistic? Autistic people will always be autistic. Autism is an important part of who we are. Trying to make your child seem less autistic will hurt them. Make sure your child doesn't get services that force them to act less autistic.

- What is the goal of the service? No service should try to make your child seem non-autistic. Good services focus on helping your child understand their autism. They help your child learn new skills. They help your child achieve their own goals.

- Who gets something good from the service? Is the service actually helping to make your child's life easier? Or is it just making your life easier? For example, some therapies could teach your child how to make eye contact. That might make your life easier when introducing your child to other people. But it would make your child's life harder. They would be forced to do something that is uncomfortable for them.

Would you use this service for a non-autistic kid? For example, imagine a service for a non-autistic child. It tells the child that they aren't allowed to talk about their favorite things. Or, imagine a service that said a non-autistic child has to hug every person they meet. There are services that treat autistic kids like this. They say autistic kids need to do things that mwake them uncomfortable. Otherwise, the autistic child is "wrong". We would be angry if non-autistic children were forced to do these things. We would be angry if non-autistic children had to hide who they are. Autistic children should get the same respect.

Think about these questions for every service you want for your child. Make sure every service provider you work with understands these ideas. You will most likely work with a team of service providers. It's important that all these providers feel the same way about helping your child. Providers should all want your child to meet your child's own goals. They should work together to help your child succeed.

If your kid was diagnosed with autism as a young child, you will probably hear the words "early intervention". This does not refer to a specific kind of service. Early intervention is the idea that getting services earlier can make a difference. It makes it quicker and easier for your child to learn new skills. It is a good idea to try and get services as soon as you can, because these services help your child!

However, some people use the words "early intervention" to mean a specific kind of service. This is called Applied Behavioral Analysis (ABA). ABA is a service that hurts autistic people. The goal of ABA is to teach autistic people to hide our autism. ABA uses rewards and punishments to train autistic people to act non-autistic. ABA therapists will often ignore autistic people when we are having a hard time. For example, an ABA therapist might only talk to an autistic child if they make eye contact. They don't care that eye contact makes that child uncomfortable. They might also punish an autistic kid for stimming or not making eye contact. They might take away the child's toys or other comfort objects.

ABA doesn't teach us the skills we actually need to succeed as autistic people. Sometimes people say they use ABA to work on other skills, like communication. But there are better ways to teach those skills, like the services we listed earlier. No autistic child needs to go through ABA. Be prepared for doctors or other people in your life to suggest ABA. Let them know you don't want that service for your child, and ask for other ideas.

Getting services that work for your child can be difficult. Some kinds of health insurance will cover ABA, but not other kinds of services. Services might not be near rural or low-income areas. Sexism and racism can also make it harder for girls and people of color to get good services. There is still a lot of work that needs to be done to make sure all autistic people can get the services that help us. There are some resources at the end of this booklet that can help you get services.

THREE

Disability and Autism

Congratulations on making it more than halfway through this booklet! You've learned a lot about autism so far. Now, we'd like to teach you more about disability.

Autism is a disability. Specifically, it is a kind of disability called a developmental disability. A developmental disability is a type of disability that starts when someone is very young. Down Syndrome and cerebral palsy are other examples of developmental disabilities.

Autism changes how we live our lives. We may learn, move, communicate, and experience the world differently. Sometimes, autism might make parts of life harder for us. That also affects how other people treat us. A lot of times, people discriminate against autistic people. Society does not try to help meet our needs. This happens to people with all kinds of disabilities.

Disability just means that someone's brain or body works very differently than most people's. Disability is a natural part of life, and disabled people have always been a part of the world.

We understand why you might not want to think that autism is a disability. Just like autism, the way our society talks about disability makes it seem like a bad and scary thing. And that's a problem! But people with disabilities are not the problem.

We may need more help with certain things than non-disabled people. But we are still an important part of society. We deserve to be treated with respect and equality.

It might be scary to be told that autism is a disability. But we're telling you because it's important that you know. Your child has rights as a person with a disability. Laws like the Americans with Disabilities Act (ADA) exist to help protect your child from discrimination.

The ADA also gives your child the right to accommodations. Accommodations are changes that make things easier for disabled people. They help us get the same chances as non-disabled people. For example, getting a sign language interpreter is an accommodation. So is getting to use headphones at school work to block out noise. Your child has the right to get what they need at school, work, and in their community. Accepting your child's disability will help you make sure they get these rights.

Your kid will feel better about themself if they grow up understanding that it's ok to have a disability. Just like there is an autistic community, there are lots of disability communities. Your child can meet other disabled people and learn to be proud of who they are. People with disabilities have worked together for many years to fight against discrimination. You and your child can join the community and help make the world a better place for disabled people!

School

Some parts of autism, like differences in communicating, will affect your child's time at school. Whether your child is already in school or will be starting school soon, it's important to think about helping them get a good education. Your child may need supports to help them learn and grow.

As a person with a disability, your child has rights at school. The law that gives your child most of these rights is called the Individuals with Disabilities Education Act, or IDEA for short. IDEA has rules for how public schools treat students with disabilities.

The IDEA says your child has the right to:

- **Get a diagnosis for their disability.** Schools have to check any child that they know or think may have a disability. This is called Child Find.

    - Even though your child might have an autism diagnosis from a doctor, the law says they also need to get one from your school.

    - The school doesn't have to give your child accommodations until they diagnose your child.

- **Get a Free and Appropriate Public Education (or FAPE for short).**

    - Your child has the right to go to school, just like all other students.

    - Your child has to get the chance to learn the same things as other students. Before IDEA, some disabled students got put in classrooms where they did not get the chance to learn anything. IDEA says this does not count as "appropriate" education.

- If your child goes to public school, the school can't charge you money for your child's services.

- **Be in the Least Restrictive Environment (or LRE for short).** This means your child should be in the same classroom as non-disabled students as much as possible.

  - The school has to try to support your child in the same classroom as everyone else. This helps make sure your child is included.

  - It makes sure your child does not automatically end up in classes that only have students with disabilities. Studies show that when students with disabilities are put in separate classrooms, they are often not treated or taught as well as when they are in classes with everyone else.

  - If you and the school agree to a separate class, the school still needs to try and include your child with non-disabled students as much as possible.

- **Get the help they need to learn.** Schools need to make a plan called an Individualized Education Plan (IEP) for each student with a disability. The IEP has to say:

  - What your child knows how to do right now

  - What your child need to learn

  - What your child's goals at school are for the next year

  - How the school will know if your child is learning

  - The services the school will give your child

  - Accommodations the school will make for your child

Schools have to work with parents to make an IEP that everyone agrees to. Parents and students have rights to make sure the IEP works for them. We have resources at the end of this booklet to help with this.

When you talk to parents or teachers about IDEA, you will hear the term "special education." Sometimes, parents think "special education" means separate classrooms or special programs for kids with disabilities. But "special education" just means services schools give kids with disabilities. "Special education" can mean supports that kids get in the same classroom as non-disabled kids. It can mean supports like speech therapy or help getting AAC. It does not just mean putting children with disabilities in a separate classroom.

IDEA applies to all public schools ("Public Education"). It also applies to charter schools. Private schools usually do not have to follow IDEA. But, sometimes a public school will pay for a child with a disability to go to a private school. If your public school district pays for your kid to go to a private school, it still has to make sure your kid gets services from IDEA.

There is one other law about your child's education rights - the Rehab Act. Section 504 is the part of the Rehab Act that talks about disability rights. You might hear it just called "504" for short. 504 says the government can't discriminate against people with disabilities. The government gives some schools money, which means those schools also have to follow the Rehab Act.

The school can make Section 504 Plans for disabled students, which say what a student needs to be able to learn. For example, the student might need:

- An iPad

- A letterboard

- Large print

- Sign language

- A support person

The accommodations your child gets from 504 plans can't change the work your child does in class too much. It also can't change too much about how the class is taught. If larger changes need to be made, then your child needs an IEP. For example:

- If your child needs to take a different test than everyone else, or not take the test at all, they probably need an IEP instead of a 504 plan.

- If your child needs an iPad to speak, but can still take the same tests as everyone else, they probably need a 504 plan.

- If your child can't do the same homework as everyone else, and needs homework that is a lot simpler, they probably need an IEP.

- If your child needs extra time to do the same homework as everyone else, but can still get it done, they probably need a 504 plan.

The Americans with Disabilities Act (ADA) is related to the Rehab Act. You might hear both 504 and ADA used when talking about your child's rights under these laws. Most private schools have to follow Section 504 because they get money from the government. Most private schools also have to follow the ADA.

We know this is a lot of information! Navigating the special education system and getting accommodations can be a confusing process. Fortunately, there are lots of parents who have been in your shoes. They have created organizations to help. Every state has at least one Parent Training and Information Center. These were made specifically to help parents understand their child's education rights, and connect them with local resources. We will have information about how to contact them at the end of this booklet.

Presuming competence in school is a big part of giving your child the best education they can get. Many parents get told by teachers that they should have low expectations for what their children can do. Having high expectations for your child makes sure that they get lots of chances to learn. They might learn differently from other kids, and they might learn at a different pace. They might need a lot of support or accommodations. But every child can learn new things. Your child has the same right to learn as any other student.

Your child has the right to be included in the same classrooms as non-disabled students. Studies show that both disabled and non-disabled students learn more when they are in the classroom together. Getting included in schools also prepares your child to be included at work and in their communities. Remember, your child has the right to an education in the least restrictive environment. If anyone tries to put your child in a separate classroom, always fight for your child to be included.

But remember that "inclusion" doesn't mean putting your child in a classroom without supports. Your child should still get the accommodations they need to do well. Some people might say the supports your child needs can't be given to them in a general education class. This has already been proven wrong by other autistic students. Supports like AAC, a 1 on 1 aide, and more have been used in classrooms together with non-disabled students.

Students with disabilities can get discriminated against in school. Trying to force your child to stay in a separate classroom from non-disabled students is one kind of discrimination. Autistic students who are also girls or people of color can face even more discrimination. Autistic girls might get diagnosed with other disorders besides autism (like anxiety disorders). They might not get offered special education services. Autistic students of color are more likely to get diagnosed with other disabilities besides autism (such as behavioral disorders). They are more likely to be put in separate classrooms, and more likely to be suspended or expelled from school.

If you think your child is getting discriminated against at school, there are people that can help. We will list some resources you can go to at the end of this booklet.

Self-advocacy

Self-advocacy means standing up for yourself. It means taking control over your own life, and fighting for your rights. Self-advocacy is very important for disabled people. All autistic people are self-advocates. We self-advocate in ways that are both big and small.

Some ways we self-advocate are by:

- Talking to other people about our disabilities

- Taking part in our IEP meetings

- Letting our work know what kind of accommodations we need

- Fighting for disability rights

Self-advocacy doesn't always look like that, though. There is no one "right" way to be a self-advocate. It's okay if your child doesn't do any of these things. They are a child! But even if you don't realize it, your child is already a self-advocate. Here are some other kinds of self-advocacy your child might already be doing:

- Saying "No!"

- Asking for help

- Telling someone to leave them alone

- Deciding what they want to do today

Your child might show self-advocacy through their behavior. Remember that behavior is one way we communicate. For example, if your child wants to get out of a loud room, they might run away if they can't let you know through words.

There are lots of ways you can support your child as they self-advocate. Here's how you can help them learn more self-advocacy skills:

- Respect when your child says they don't want to do something. If it is something they absolutely have to do, take the time to explain why. Try to get them involved in figuring out how to make the situation easier for them.

- Help your child learn to communicate in ways that work for them. Self-advocacy can be through behavior. But your child's life (and yours!) will be easier if they have other ways to show how they feel. Helping your child communicate helps them self-advocate more easily.

- Respect your child's boundaries. Never force your child to touch or make eye contact with another person. Setting boundaries is an important part of self-advocacy. Even if it is a family member, if your child is uncomfortable hugging that person, they should not have to.

- Give your child choices about their everyday life. This can be as simple as letting them choose their own clothes, food, or hobbies they will explore.

- Make sure your child is involved in decision-making about their life. For example, bring your child to their IEP meetings. Explain what is going on, and ask for their opinion.

- Help your child meet autistic adults, so they have strong role models.

Respecting your child's wants and needs is important for any child, but especially for an autistic child. Society often takes away choices for people with disabilities. For example, we may get placed in separate classrooms from non-disabled kids. We might get told we can't do things, for unfair reasons. Self-advocacy is an important skill to build your child. It teaches them that they have the right to make their own decisions, and that those decisions deserve to be respected.

Who do I tell about my child's autism?

One of the first people you should tell about your child's autism is your child! Your child has the right to know this important information about their life. Your child probably already knows that they think and act differently from most other children. Learning about autism helps them know why, and helps them be proud of who they are.

Your autistic child has a lot to be proud of! There are many role models in the autistic community that they can look up to. Here is a list of just a few famous autistic people:

- Temple Grandin – Animal Scientist

- Dan Aykroyd – Comedic Actor

- Chris Rock – Actor & Comedian

- Kodi Lee – Musician

- Susan Boyle – Singer

- Stephen Wiltshire - Artist

- Daryl Hannah – Actress & Environmental Activist

- Armani Williams – Racecar Driver

- Sir Anthony Hopkins – Actor

- Hannah Gadsby - Comedian

- Kalin Bennett – Division I College basketball player

- Silvia Moreno-Garcia - Author

There are many resources on how to tell children from different age groups and reading levels that they are autistic. We have some recommendations at the end of this booklet. You could also use a social story to explain autism to your child.

Just like any other child, parenting an autistic child can be frustrating. But you should never talk about autism in a bad way to your child. So, it is good to have a family member or close friend that you can talk to who understands your child's diagnosis. But they need to respect your child's privacy if you share difficult things.

Not everyone you talk to about autism will understand. Our society says a lot of bad things about autism. Sometimes, your friends and family might believe those things. Other times, they might just not know much about autism. Or, they might have different ideas about what autism means. For example, some cultures think eye contact is very important. Other cultures do not think it is important, or even find it rude. Depending on your culture, your community might react differently to your autistic child not making eye contact. Also, like we said earlier, doctors are less likely to diagnose autistic people of color. If your family belongs to a community that doctors diagnose less, your community might not get as much information about autism.

In general, it should be your child's choice to decide who they tell about their autism. Some doctors, service providers, or teachers might need to know about your child's autism when they are young. But whether or not someone is autistic, and what autism is like for them, is personal information. If you teach your child to be proud of being autistic, they will be more likely to want to tell people about it! But your child should always have control over the information about their life. Choosing when to share that we are autistic is another form of self-advocacy.

Putting it all together

Autism is a big part of what makes your child who they are. Your child might need different supports than their non-autistic peers. They might think about and process the world in a different way. But your child is the same kid you have always known and loved. Part of being a parent is learning to see the world from your child's point of view. That helps you figure out how to best support them as they grow. That means loving and accepting your child as their entire autistic self. We hope this booklet helped you begin to learn more about autism and how to help your child succeed.

Remember that you're not alone! There are lots of autistic adults who can tell you more about what being autistic means to them. There are online resources from parents who have been in your shoes. There are also state and local resources to help you and your child find support. You have already taken an important first step by reading this booklet! As you learn more about autism, you will feel more confident.

You and your child have a great future ahead of you.

FOUR

Resources

You can also find links to these resources at
autisticadvocacy.org/resources/books/start-here-resources

Books

Welcome to the Autistic Community - by the Autistic Self Advocacy Network. Also available online at <u>autismacceptance.com</u>

Sincerely, Your Autistic Child: What People on the Autism Spectrum Wish Their Parents Knew About Growing Up, Acceptance, and Identity - by Autistic Women & Nonbinary Network

Uniquely Human: A Different Way of Seeing Autism - by Barry Prizant

The Real Experts: Readings for Parents of Autistic Children (anthology)

Loud Hands: Autistic People, Speaking (anthology)

All the Weight of our Dreams: on living racialized autism (anthology)

Spectrums: Autistic Transgender People in their Own Words (anthology)

Typed Words, Loud Voices: A Collection (anthology)

Why Johnny Doesn't Flap: NT is OK! - by Clay and Gail Morton

Media for kids

Just Right for You - by Melanie Heyworth

All Cats Are On The Autism Spectrum - by Kathy Hoopmann

I Like Dinosaurs Too! - by Mandy Farmer

Tomas Loves...: A rhyming book about fun, friendship - and autism - by Jude Welton

Autistic Legends Alphabet Book - by Beck Feiner

Sesame Street - A television show with an autistic character, Julia.

Loop - A Pixar animated short film featuring a non-speaking autistic girl of color.

Documentaries & movies for parents

Intelligent Lives - A documentary that follows the lives of 3 young adults with intellectual disabilities. https://intelligentlives.org/

The Reason I Jump - A documentary following 5 autistic young adults.

LISTEN: A short film made by and with nonspeaking autistic people https://communicationfirst.org/listen/

In A Beat - A short film about an autistic teen of color. https://www.youtube.com/watch?v=WBlge8kXdR0&vl=en

Federally-funded programs

Parent Training and Information Centers (PTIs) and Community Parent Resource Centers (CPRCs) can help you navigate the special education system. Find your PTI by going to https://www.parentcenterhub.org/find-your-center/

If your child is being discriminated against, your Protection & Advocacy Agency (P&A) might be able to help. P&As help people with disabilities fight for our rights, and make sure states follow disability laws. There is a P&A in every state. You can find the P&A in your state by going to https://www.ndrn. org/about/ndrn-member-agencies/

Every state also has a Developmental Disabilities Council (DD Council). These are groups that advocate for the rights of people with developmental disabilities. They believe that disabled people should be the main people to have a say in laws that affect their lives. It's required that some members of the councils be people with disabilities themselves. DD Council meetings could be a good chance for your child to learn more about self-advocacy. They could meet potential mentors from the self-advocacy movement. Find your state DD Council by going to https://acl.gov/programs/aging-and-disability-networks/state-councils-developmental-disabilities

The National Resource Center for Supported Decision-Making has information about supported decision-making in each state. http://www.supporteddecisionmaking.org/

Parenting blogs/resources

Thinking Person's Guide to Autism - Blogs written by a variety of autistic people and parents of autistic children. www.Thinkingautismguide.com

We Are Like Your Child - Blogs written by autistic adults to show how we felt and acted as children, and show that your autistic child may act the same way and still become a happy and self-determined adult. https://wearelikeyourchild.blogspot.com/

Ollibean - A community of parents, families and disability advocates that puts out blogs and other information about autism acceptance. www.Ollibean.com

Autistikids - A collection of blogs and resources for parents of autistic children. www.Autistikids.com

Reframing Autism - An Australian autistic advocacy group. https://www.reframingautism.com.au/

Sesame Street and Autism - A resource that includes videos and articles for parents and kids, that are also available in Spanish. https://autism.sesamestreet.org/

Advocacy organizations

Little Lobbyists - Advocates for children with disabilities and complex medical needs. www.littlelobbyists.org

Autistic Self Advocacy Network - Advocates for autistic people to be included in all aspects of society, and have our voices heard in policy discussions. They also have Affiliate Groups throughout the U.S. and internationally for autistic people to join the self-advocacy movement. www.autisticadvocacy.org

The Arc - Advocates for people with intellectual and developmental disabilities. They also provide services for people with disabilities. They have chapters across the United States for people to get involved in disability advocacy. www.thearc.org

Self Advocates Becoming Empowered (SABE) - The United State's national self-advocacy organization. They have chapters, called People First groups, across the country. https://www.sabeusa.org/

Communication

Communication First - A nonprofit whose mission is "to educate the public, advocate for policy reform, and engage the judicial system to advance the rights, autonomy, opportunity, and dignity of people with speech-related communication disabilities and conditions." https://communicationfirst.org/

Everybody Communicates: A Toolkit for Accessing Communication Assessments, Funding, and Accommodations - https://odpc.ucsf.edu/communications-paper

Assistiveware's Learn AAC Guide - https://www.assistiveware.com/learn-aac/learn-aac-guide

Penn State Literacy Instruction - A website that gives guidelines for teaching reading skills to learners who use AAC. https://aacliteracy.psu.edu/

Resources for disabilities that many autistic people have

National Center for Learning Disabilities - A nonprofit that "improves the lives of the 1 in 5 with learning and attention issues by empowering parents and young adults, transforming schools, and advocating for equal rights and opportunities." https://www.ncld.org/

Children and Adults with Attention-Deficit/Hyperactivity Disorder (CHADD) - A nonprofit whose mission is to improve the lives of people with ADHD. https://chadd.org/

National Down Syndrome Congress - A nonprofit organization whose mission is to improve the world for people with Down Syndrome. https://www.ndsccenter.org/

Resources on race and gender in the autistic community

Autistic Women & Nonbinary Network (AWN) -Works to provide community, support, and resources for Autistic women, girls, nonbinary people, and all others of marginalized genders. www.awnnetwork.org

Autism and Race - Curates a list of blogs and resources for autistic people of color and their families. Runs the Autistic People of Color Fund. https://autismandrace.com/